WEIGHT LOSS

Proven ways to lose weight without dieting

JENNY HORTON

Table of contents

INTRODUCTION

When it comes to shedding excess fat, it goes without saying that dieting can help you shed excess pounds. You find it difficult to hold back or stick to a strict diet. Luckily, there are some proven ways to lose weight without dieting. Certain changes need to be made. However, instead of addressing the mental health issues of dieting by eating less, you lose weight by increasing activity, changing meal times, and using certain tricks to boost your metabolism. Using these tricks together can lead to significant weight loss. Here are eight proven ways to lose weight without dieting.

CHAPTER ONE

Do cardio in the morning before eating

Aerobic exercises such as running, biking, and climbing stairs can do wonders when it comes to burning calories and reducing body fat. People who avoid diets probably don't want to embark on a rigorous exercise routine, but doing a short cardio workout before a meal can yield amazing results. A study published in the British Journal of Nutrition found that people who did cardio in the morning (that is, before meals) while fasting burned 20% more fat than those who ate beforehand. I understand. This is because when your body is sober, it burns fat instead of carbs for energy. So you can get amazing results in just 20 minutes of your morning workout.

Sleep more

Even if you don't want to cut back on your calorie intake or increase your physical activity, you can still lose a few extra pounds just by working on your sleep patterns. Not getting enough sleep can make you feel tired all day long, but it can also cause you to gain fat. In her 2010 study published in the Annals of Internal Medicine, the subject found that just by increasing her sleep time by three hours, he burned 400 calories a night. Additionally, subjects who slept 8.5 hours each night lost 60% less muscle mass than those who slept 5.5 hours each night, and the extra sleep helped boost metabolism.

Drink more water

Another proven way to lose weight without a strict diet is to drink more water. Some people worry about drinking more water because the extra weight in water can increase the number on the scale. You will burn more fat. Additionally, her 2013 study, published in the Journal of Clinical and Diagnostic Research, found that a girl who drank 500ml of water before each meal lost weight without further diet changes. , found that the body mass index decreased. Therefore, be sure to drink 0.5 liters of water before each meal to boost your metabolism and reduce hunger.

CHAPTER TWO

Eat more protein

Increasing your protein intake is one of the best ways to boost your metabolism and lose weight. A 2008 study in the American Journal of Clinical Nutrition found that protein helps increase satiety, reduce hunger, and naturally reduce calorie intake. It's also great for building muscle and leads to more fat loss. Luckily, you don't have to change your entire diet to get more protein. Many people see positive effects just by drinking a few proteins shakes each day. You may want to improve your results by eating a high-protein breakfast to help you feel full.

Try intermittent fasting

Dieting is not the only way to burn excess fat. Interestingly, even if you eat a lot of calories each day, you can lose weight as long as you eat each meal in a short time. This is known as intermittent fasting, and many athletes do it. I swear Intermittent fasting usually involves eating all of your daily meals within

8 hours, fasting for the remaining 16 hours, and then eating again. It turns into fat storage, reduces your fat mass, and ultimately loses weight. However, overeating during the diet period should be avoided.

CHAPTER THREE

Avoid stress and anxiety

Daily stress and high levels of anxiety can be incredibly counterproductive for those trying to lose weight. If you are not careful, you can easily overeat. Luckily, there are some natural ways to manage stress and anxiety. Exercise is a great way to de-stress and lose weight at the same time. Getting at least 8 hours of sleep each night also makes a big difference. You should also avoid everyday stressors. For example, if your daily commute is stressful, try walking or biking instead.

Lift weights regularly

If you're not a fan of dieting, resistance training is one of the best ways to keep your body in shape. It helps. For every pound of muscle, you gain, your body burns more calories, even when you're resting. It also has other benefits. For example, when you lift weights, much of the food you eat is used to repair and rebuild your body. This means you can build muscle while losing fat. People who lift weights are often able to eat more than they normally would while maintaining or losing weight.

Increase Vitamin D Levels

Various vitamins and minerals can help keep your body in shape and help you lose weight, but vitamin D is arguably the most important. Many people suffer from vitamin D deficiency, which often leads to metabolic syndrome, depression, and anxiety, all of which contribute to weight gain. It's also surprisingly easy to boost your vitamin D levels. Spending 30 minutes in the sun every day is a natural way to boost your vitamin D levels. Certain beverages such as fortified orange juice and other foods are also high in vitamin D. You can also take a vitamin D supplement to keep your vitamin D levels high.

CHAPTER FOUR

Conclusion

The fastest and most effective way to lose weight is to combine a healthy diet with a good exercise routine, but you can try these effective options without dieting. Whether you're fasting, drinking more water, or simply wanting to get more sleep, all of these can contribute to weight loss.

Of course, you should try as many of these tips together as possible for the best results. You'll soon find it much easier to lose weight. However, if you eat too much, you are likely to gain weight, so be careful.

www.ingramcontent.com/pod-product-compliance
Lightning Source LLC
LaVergne TN
LVHW020547160826
845677LV00015B/4254
9798352898727